THE BEGINNER'S GUIDE TO
OIL PULLING
nature's therapy

LEARN HOW TO HEAL YOUR BODY
BY USING AN ANCIENT ORAL
DETOX THERAPY

KATE EVANS SCOTT
DAVID PEARSON

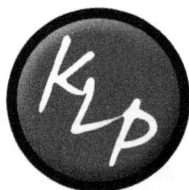

KL PRESS

DISCLAIMER

No part of this publication may be reproduced or transmitted in any form or by any means, mechanical or electronic, including photocopying or recording, or by any information storage and retrieval system, or transmitted by email without permission in writing from the publisher.

Although the author and publisher have made every effort to ensure that the information in this book was correct at press time, the author and publisher do not assume and hereby disclaim any liability to any party for any loss, damage, or disruption caused by errors or omissions, whether such errors or omissions result from negligence, accident, or any other cause.

This book is not intended as a substitute for the medical advice of physicians. The reader should regularly consult a physician in matters relating to his/her health and particularly with respect to any symptoms that may require diagnosis or medical attention.

This book is dedicated to everyone who seeks to live their healthiest life.

ACKNOWLEDGMENTS

Thank You to our friends and family for your encouragement. Your support has been the cornerstone of this creative process.

A special thanks also goes out to you the reader ~ we are grateful to be sharing this journey to health and happiness together with you.

CONTENTS

CHAPTER 1

CHAPTER 2

CHAPTER 3

CONTENTS

CHAPTER 4

CHAPTER 5

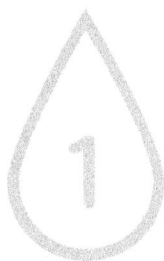

OIL PULLING: NEW DISCOVERY OF AN ANCIENT HEALTH SECRET

WHAT IS OIL PULLING?

Oil pulling sounds like a term you might find alongside "oil fracking" in an article about the country's fuel oil resources. However, oil pulling and oil fracking couldn't be further from each other.

Oil pulling is a simple, natural process that has been used for thousands of years to improve oral health, prevent illness, and increase longevity. The process involves swishing high grade oils (such as coconut oil or sesame oil) in your mouth for twenty minutes each day, and then spitting. It's as simple as that, and it claims to address all of these ailments with one simple practice:

- Acne and skin dryness
- Allergies (seasonal and other)
- Arthritis
- Bronchitis
- Constipation
- Chronic Fatigue
- Colitis
- Crohn's Disease
- Chronic Headaches
- Dental Caries and Cavities
- Dermatitis
- Diabetes
- Eczema
- Gingivitis
- Hemorrhoids
- Hypertension
- Insomnia
- Migraine Headaches
- Peptic Ulcers
- Premenstrual Syndrome
- Periodontal Disease
- Sinusitis
- Tooth Abscesses

The anti-inflammatory properties of the oils may also indicate that oil pulling would be an effective method in dealing with such ailments as heart disease, stroke, infertility, nerve disorders, psychiatric disorders, and much more.

This "miracle cure" is called oil pulling because the oil is pulling toxins out of your body from all the little spaces in your mouth that your tooth brush (and even your mouthwash) can't possibly reach. Oil pulling has made its way out of the traditional cultures and into mainstream media, catching its few minutes of fame even on major network news channels and hitting the blogosphere like wildfire.

But is it just hype, or is there scientific truth behind this strange and new alternative health craze? We'll figure all of that out, but first let's get familiar with the process and explore its deep roots in medical history.

THE PROCESS

Just swish, spit, and heal. It's as easy as that? Maybe not. Have you ever tried to swish around a cheek full of mouthwash for longer than a few minutes? Yeah, it's not that easy. In this process, a tablespoon of oil needs to be swished for at least *fifteen minutes a day* to achieve its highly acclaimed health benefits.

But don't worry, with practice, the swishing and swilling process of oil pulling will start coming naturally. Here's a tip for starters so you don't get frustrated right off the bat: Remember to swish constantly, but not necessarily *vigorously*. The idea is not to give your cheeks, jaws, and tongue a workout. Instead, the process should be relaxing and enjoyable... definitely not strenuous or aggravating, because then you won't do it.

RISE, SHINE, AND RELAX

Oil pulling should be practiced first thing in the morning on an empty stomach, preferably in a comfortable sitting position with your chin tilted slightly upward. This is a meditative, ergonomic posture that will help your body and mind relax, allowing the system to focus on detoxification, and the empty stomach is crucial to the detox process.

Taking that few minutes to meditate (sit quietly) while swishing each day reduces stress, which has all kinds of positive effects on your physical and mental well-being including increased heart, digestive, and mental health. So think of this as your swish-meditation! It's a health double-whammy.

But honestly, if you have to swish while you take a shower, get dressed, and pack your kids' backpacks... no-one's judging. Do what you have to do. You're still going to get health benefits from the oil pulling process.

TAKE A LOVIN' SPOONFUL

Of oil, that is. Sitting in this meditative position, take one tablespoon of high quality oil (like organic cold pressed coconut, sesame, sunflower, olive, or other) into your mouth. Swish it between your teeth, sucking and pulling to move the oil through as many spaces as possible, reaching as much tooth and gum tissue as possible. Swish the oil back and forth between your cheeks and roll it over and under your tongue. Do this for 15 – 20 minutes.

SPIT AND RINSE

When the oil has become white, milky, and thin, you're ready to spit. It's really important that you do not swallow the oil because at this point, it has already pulled out all of that bacteria and numerous toxins which are floating around inside the saliva. Swallowing would dump all that junk right back into your system. You really don't want to do that.

Spit into the sink and then rinse either with purified water or salt water. Brush your teeth and floss as usual. Remember that oil pulling is complimentary to your regular oral care routine, but should not replace brushing and flossing.

THE REASON OIL PULLING WORKS

At this point, you might be asking yourself how in the world this all works. Like many people out there, when it comes to your health, you need a rational explanation. Well, for all of you smart data-gatherers out there, here's the science behind the swish.

PLAQUE MAKES POCKETS

Plaque is that thin yellow film of mucus, bacteria, and food that builds up at the base of your teeth. It's full of all kinds of organisms including parasites, pesticides, food additives, and bacteria. Yuck, right? It happens to the best of us. Actually, it happens to all of us. We do our best to brush, floss, and rinse it away. But no matter how hard you try, you can't reach the little pockets beneath the gums caused by plaque. Nope, not even with floss. Okay, there are these pockets. So, what?

BACTERIA PARTIES

What's going on in these tiny pockets is a little bacteria party.... And not the fun kind, even though there might be cake. Yep, the pockets under the gum line fill with tiny bacterium. Up to 100 million different bacteria at any given time are having a party in your mouth. These miniscule pocket parties are full of exotoxins and endotoxins that slide right down into your digestive tract every time you swallow.

These bacteria and toxins are the cause of bloody, swollen gums (gingivitis) and bad breath (halitosis), and they're also the jumping point for a host of other health complications.

OIL PICKS THE POCKETS

Why doesn't floss get the bacteria out? Why doesn't brushing with tooth paste crash that party? Why can't mouthwash do its job and wash it all away? Because none of these things are viscous. They're not "sticky" like oil. The oil stretches and thins as you swish it, reaching up into each of those miniscule pockets, glomming onto the toxins, and yanking them back out.

Actually, the toxins often glom onto the fatty content of the oils, because many harmful toxins and bacteria are fat-soluble. You can swish and slosh as much water as you want and they won't budge. But give them a drip of oil and they're as good as gone.

When you spit and rinse after swishing around that nice fatty oil, you flush all of those harmful toxins right down the sink (or toilet, or wastebasket... wherever you spit). But here's the thing... it's not a one-time cleanse. Every time you eat or drink anything but purified water, you're building up plaque and tucking more toxins into pockets. It's an inevitable part of being alive.

You absolutely must repeat this process (Rise and Shine, Lovin' Spoonful, Swish, Spit and Rinse) every morning in order to continue to reap the benefits of this simple detoxification. You can start by trying it for forty-five days. Within the first two months, most people see a remarkable difference in the whiteness of their teeth, gingivitis is completely cleared up, and bad breath is gone.

Many other minor maladies from headaches to joint pain, eczema to digestive sensitivity, mysteriously disappear within this two-month "trial" period. *Well, maybe not so mysteriously.* There's real science to back up the validity of this ancient Ayurvedic practice. Keep reading and you'll begin to understand how and why it works. It's all about balance... and organs, and toxins, and tongues. Oh, my!

BEST OILS USED IN OIL PULLING

It's always best to use organic, unrefined, cold pressed oils for oil-pulling because these will not contain any chemical residues. They are the purest form of oil, and when you're trying to take out toxins, it's important not to be putting new toxins in.

Which organic, unrefined, cold pressed oil you use may just be a matter of preference and your intentions for oil-pulling. Some of the most commonly used oils are sesame, coconut, and olive while occasionally people use safflower and sunflower oils.

Just remember that when we specify oils below, we are talking about unrefined, cold-pressed, organic food grade oils.

SESAME OIL

There's a reason that sesame oil has been used by healers for centuries. In fact, there are a lot of reasons. It has incredible healing properties. Sesame oil is a natural

antiviral and **antifungal** agent, and is specifically good for targeting staphylococcus (staph infections) and streptococcus (strep).

Sesame oil also has fantastic **antioxidant** properties. Once it penetrates the skin, which it does quickly, the sesame oil rapidly neutralizes free oxygen radicals. The oil becomes a "sweeper," helping your immune system keep everything in check.

Free oxygen radicals are your body's evil wild card. They're unhitched atoms that need to grab onto an electron from another molecule to survive. In the fraction of a second that constitutes their short existence, free radicals can start of a chain reaction of oxidation that can leave serious damage in your body. Left unchecked due to a tapped-out or otherwise unhealthy immune system, this oxidation process causes clogged arteries and destruction of DNA and could potentially play a role in the growth of cancer cells, stroke, and heart disease.

If swishing with an inexpensive oil has all of these positive health effects, and no side effects, there's absolutely no reason not to try it!

COCONUT OIL

Coconut oil has been getting its due credit in the world of health and wellness over the past few years. With an abundance of coconut products hitting the shelves, from coconut water to coconut yogurt, we can't ignore the fact that there's something good about this simple tree nut.

Just like sesame oil, coconut oil has **antioxidant, antibacterial,** and **antiviral** properties that help heal and prevent some of the most common ailments. The use of coconut oil has also been associated with **weight loss** due to the way the medium chain triglycerides (MCT) in coconut oil are metabolized. Increasing your consumption of MCT fats like coconut oil will keep you feeling fuller, longer while increasing your energy levels.[1, 2]

Because of its simple composition, coconut oil is quickly absorbed through the skin. That means all of its nutritive properties go straight into your bloodstream and are put right to work helping to increase **cardiovascular health, cognitive function, bone and join health,** and aid in the **detoxification of vital organs.**

Did you think coconut oil was bad for you because it's almost all fat? Well, that's what the soy and corn oil marketing managers wanted you think. Back in the early sixties, they launched a campaign attacking coconut oil in favor of their products... but now their strategy is being debunked by all sorts of academic research.

In fact, there are populations of people in the South Pacific that eat the highest dietary percentage of coconut (meat, milk, oil) in the world, and 60% of their diet comes from this type of saturated fat. These are some of the healthiest people on the planet. They suffer from absolutely no cardiovascular disease at all. [3]

If you need another reason to use coconut oil, you can follow your taste buds! Coconut oil has a mild, sweet flavor that is pleasant to the palate. This is important because if you don't like the flavor of the oil, you are unlikely to continue oil pulling long-term.

OLIVE OIL

Some people may use olive oil for pulling simply because it's readily available, and is often already in their cupboards for cooking. However, olive oil has a host of health benefits that are utilized when it's swished in the oral cavity.

The high polyphenol count in cold pressed extra virgin olive oil makes it an incredibly powerful **anti-inflammatory** agent and **antioxidant.** Current research also shows that the use of extra virgin olive oil can decrease the risks for certain types of cancer (especially stomach cancer), lower LDL cholesterol levels, and prevent cardiovascular disease. [4]

The problem with olive oil for oil pulling is the flavor. I know, we shouldn't let our taste buds get in the way of optimal health. But let's get real. If it tastes horrible we're not going to keep doing it. If you happen to love the taste of olive oil, then by all means, go ahead and reap all of these wonderful benefits. But if you want something with a slightly milder taste, go with coconut or sunflower oil.

SUNFLOWER OIL

Along with sesame oil, sunflower oil has been a mainstay in the Ayurvedic practice of oil pulling for centuries. Its health properties are similar to sesame and coconut oil, plus it's **rich in vitamin E**, which helps keep cells hydrated and skin feeling soft. [5]

Sunflower oil also **decreases your risk for developing heart disease, lowers cholesterol,** and **reduces incidence of arthritis and asthma.** With its mild flavor and long shelf-life, sunflower oil is the first choice for many people choosing to incorporate oil pulling into their health care routine.

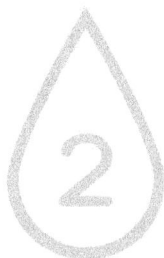

HISTORY OF OIL PULLING IN AYURVEDIC MEDICINE

AYURVEDA: THE PRACTICE AND ORIGIN

Ayurveda is a traditional medical practice that has been used effectively in India for thousands of years. As early as 3,000 – 5,000 years ago, Ayurvedic healers were prescribing oil pulling with sesame or sunflower oil as a cure or preventative medicine for infectious diseases and chronic conditions.

Often called the mother of medical science, the first written reference to Ayurveda occurs in the oldest book currently on record, the Veda, which literally means "knowledge." The book is separated into four sections: Rigveda, Yajurveda, Samaveda, and Atharvaveda. Ayurveda is part of the Atharvaveda. Ayur means "life," and so the section of the Vedas that imparts medical advice is literally translated as "life knowledge."

Ayurveda heavily influenced the early medical practices of Chinese, Tibetan, and Greek cultures. In some senses, you can see the similarity between the Hindu or yogic system's use of chakras (healing, energy points in the body) and the Ayurvedic belief that everything is connected.

Aptly named, this system of medical practice is completely different from the medicine we practice in the west. It is based on the innate knowledge that not only are the mind and body connected, but so are the mind and body inherently linked to the soul and to nature. In order to be healthy, all aspects of being must be in balance and working symbiotically to create a peaceful (healthy) existence.

Ayurvedic medicine is highly individualized based on each person's body or constitutional type, called *prakruti*. This system takes into account an individual's DNA, as well the environmental factors surrounding them, in order to prescribe a treatment that will best suit their specific needs at that specific point in time. This system understands how each individual will react differently to various treatments and environmental factors based on their *prakruti* type.[6]

An Ayurvedic practitioner will then take that initial assessment and prescribe various healing methods, the focus being mainly on herbal remedies and preventatives, as well as nutrition, meditation, massage, and moderate exercise.

While western medicine generally looks at Ayurveda as a complimentary or alternative medicine, traditional medical practice like Ayurveda provides the primary health care for up to 80% of the population of some Asian an African countries. Over the course of the past decade, people in developed countries with access to western medicine have also begun to take advantage of the natural path offered by traditional medicine.[7]

OIL PULLING IN AYURVEDIC MEDICINE

Called Kaval or Gandush in Sanskrit, the practice of holding or swishing oil in the mouth has been used to effectively cure over thirty systemic diseases for thousands of years, and the simple treatment essentially remains the same today. [8]

Originally, Ayurvedic practitioners used sesame oil because it was considered a gift from the gods due to its incredible health properties. It was also a readily available, inexpensive oil with a pleasant flavor... and it still is!

The portion of the Veda that addressed dentistry and oral health, the Schalakya, demonstrates several different methods of using oils for healing specific ailments. One involves filling the mouth completely with oil and then spitting. The other involves holding oil in the mouth for a few minutes, gargling, and then spitting.

Oil pulling, the act of swishing the oil between the teeth and around the oral cavity, is a process that has been recently "rediscovered" by modern practitioners. However, this simple process has already been used for thousands of years to effectively treat such ailments as headaches, migraines, diabetes, and asthma as well as oral maladies like dry mouth and throat, tooth decay, halitosis, and cracked lips.

The modern version of oil pulling was instituted by a Ukrainian physician by the name of Dr. F. Karach in the early 1990's. Dr. Karach claimed that the technique could cure a number of ailments from hormonal imbalance to cracked lips... and that it had already given him relief from his own chronic blood condition and his painful arthritis. The efficacy of oil pulling on oral health is perhaps easy to understand, but swishing oil to cure arthritis? How can that possibly work?

Ayurvedic medicine correlates the tongue to various bodily functions and organs. Remember, Ayurveda is a holistic approach to medicine—everything is connected! Practitioners can look at the tongue to diagnose diseases within these organs, and also cleanse the tongue as treatment for diseases. Specific areas of the tongue are directly linked to health of the spleen, heart, lungs, liver, stomach, pancreas, and kidneys. [9]

As previously explained, oil pulling extracts toxins from the tongue, gums, teeth, and oral cavity, breaks them down in the saliva, and expresses them from the body. Detoxifying the tongue in this way has a restorative effect on the associated organs and functions.

KATE EVANS SCOTT & DAVID PEARSON

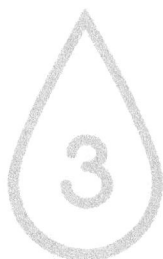

OIL PULLING FOR ORAL HEALTH

The most obvious and immediate effect of oil pulling on one's health and wellness is in the mouth, although the condition of your teeth and gums are often either a predictor or a cause of ailments elsewhere in the body. Clean, white teeth and pale pink gums that do not bleed when brushing are a good indicator of a healthy body. Wherein yellowed, cracked teeth and puffy, red gums can point to other serious health issues from cardiac disease to kidney failure.

But let's get back to where it all starts, the mouth. For many people, oil pulling can whiten teeth and strengthen gums within just a few weeks of incorporating the twenty-minute swish into their daily routine. In some cases, results are much quicker—even within as little as ten days! [10] Because the oil is viscous, it reaches up into places that neither the tooth brush nor the floss can reach, pulling out the nasty bacteria and toxins left behind by these more popular methods of oral care.

Sometimes the instant gratification (almost) of seeing results in your smile is enough to commit you to the practice long-term, when you'll start seeing even deeper effects on your health. Just don't stop when your teeth get whiter and your gums are a nice pale pink. Keep going for a few weeks to see how the practice can bring balance to the rest of your body.

OIL PULLING FOR HEALTHY TEETH

Oil pulling is a simple practice that not only prevents tooth decay, but can actually reverse it! That doesn't quite seem possible, does it? Modern dentistry tells us that the only way to treat a cavity is to dig it out and fill it, but there's another way.

Here's what's going on in your mouth at any given moment:[11] Your teeth are coated with a thin film of plaque, which is mostly made up of bacteria. That bacteria feeds on the sugar in sweets and starches. When the bacteria gets plenty of sugar to feed on, they create an abundance of acid. The acid eats away at the tooth enamel, sucking out the minerals and leaving a big old hole in your tooth. So, when your dentist tells you not to munch pretzels and suck on hard candy all day, this is why! Those foods literally set off a food chain that leaves holes in your teeth.

Your saliva is actually the good guy in this story. Saliva is what's trying to wash away the bacteria and

KATE EVANS SCOTT & DAVID PEARSON

neutralize the acid. When you see a little white spot on your tooth, that's the start of the decay process. It's probably something your dentist is going to "watch," but not do much about except to prescribe fluoride and tell you to keep brushing until there's an actual hole in the tooth enamel that he or she can scrape out and fill.

Adding oil pulling to your daily brushing routine can actually help your saliva grab onto that bacteria (because bacteria loves to latch onto fats) and suck it away, stopping the acid attack on the white spot. Then, minerals from saliva and the healing properties of these oils can begin to re-mineralize that weak spot on the tooth. Re-mineralization means "healing" to the tooth enamel.

While researchers are still studying the efficacy of oil pulling and its implications on western dental care practices, there are countless stories from people who have tried oil-pulling to combat cavities, demonstrating in a very tangible way that it does indeed work!

"My doctor noticed white spots on two of my teeth during a regular dental exam," says Mindy, 37, of Michigan. "He prescribed me a fluoride rinse that was supposed to help re-mineralize my teeth, but I didn't want to use fluoride. After doing some research on healing tooth decay naturally, I started oil-pulling. When I went back to the dentist at my six-month checkup, the decay was gone! My dentist told me that the fluoride worked, and he was completely floored when I told him that I hadn't used it!"

There are numerous stories of people like Mindy who have reversed the decay process in less than forty-five days with a simple daily oil pulling practice added to their regular dental health regime.

OIL PULLING FOR HALITOSIS

Halitosis. In layman's terms, that's bad breath. Halitosis is usually caused by issues in the oral cavity like gingivitis and periodontitis, but can also be rooted in and indicative of serious health issues like diabetes. Whatever the cause, halitosis stems from harmful anaerobic bacteria in the mouth.

Researchers from the Meenakshi Ammal Dental College in Chennai, India and the Narayana Dental College in Nellore, Tamil Nadu, India studied the efficacy of oil pulling in reducing symptoms of chronic halitosis.[12] In the study, they used Chlorhexidine mouth wash as the control because it is considered the gold standard in anticavity and gingivitis-reducing properties, reducing mouth odor by 69% and tongue odor by 78% after just one week of use.

What the researchers found is quite astonishing: That oil pulling with sesame oil was just as effective in reducing mouth and tongue odor as Chlorhexidine.

This is a promising find, because oil used in pulling is six times more cost effective than Chlorhexidine and is readily available in most households... even in developing countries where other dental care practices might be out of reach.

Bad breath is not a laughing matter. In fact, halitosis can really be a crippling social disease and is also indicative of other health problems. Oil pulling heals the halitosis, it isn't just masking bad breath like a mint or breath spray would. It's addressing the root cause of the bad breath, and thus also pulling the rest of the body into balance.

OIL PULLING FOR GUM HEALTH

Healthy gums not only make for a prettier smile, they are also an indicator that all is well in your body. Gingivitis is a swelling or inflammation of the gums often indicated by bloody bristles when brushing or red-pink spit after flossing. Gingivitis is a periodontal disease that destroys

KATE EVANS SCOTT & DAVID PEARSON

the tissues supporting the teeth such as the gums, ligaments, and tooth sockets. Gingivitis not only causes "loose teeth" and puffy gums, it can also lead to tooth decay.[13]

Gingivitis has a number of causes, including systemic diseases, infections, untreated diabetes, pregnancy, poor dental hygiene, misaligned teeth, orthodontics, and use of some medications.

In a 2009 report, researchers studied a group of adolescent boys with plaque-induced gingivitis. The data revealed that oil pulling reduced the plaque index and modified gingival scores of the group that incorporated oil pulling into their oral care routine. Furthermore, they discovered that the count of aerobic microorganisms in the plaque was remarkably reduced.[14] This means that there were less sugar-eating bacteria present on the teeth of the study group, the kind of bacteria that thrive on starches and turn food into acid.

A reduction in sugar-eating bacteria indicates a potential reduction in cavities as well as a restorative effect on the gums.

Predating the 2009 study, research results of a 2007 study were published in the *Journal of Oral Health and Community Dentistry (JOHCD)* that clearly indicated the efficacy of incorporating oil pulling into the normal oral care routine. [15] Test subjects showed significantly reduced signs of gingivitis after 45 days of oil pulling with sunflower oil.

It has clearly been demonstrated that oil pulling helps to eliminate the gum disease and cavities that are likely the symptom another bodily imbalance, but through the detox process and the oil's restorative properties, oil pulling may also be helping to heal the deeper-rooted issue ultimately resulting in the gingivitis and decay.

OIL PULLING FOR DENTAL PAIN AND LOOSE TEETH

While there really have been no substantial scientific studies on the effects of oil pulling on dental pain and loose teeth, there is a mounting database of anecdotal evidence pointing to the success people have had using the procedure to treat tooth pain and to root teeth that were loose in their sockets. These testimonies can't be taken lightly when considering the indication for such healing attributed to oil pulling in the thousands-years old Veda scriptures.

What worked thousands of years ago, works today.

According to Oilpulling.com, an authoritative voice and advocate for oil pulling and Ayurvedic medicine on the web, Dr. Karach, the "re-inventor" of the modern oil pulling practice, says this about its efficacy. "[Oil pulling] is analgesic in relieving pain, antibiotic in eliminating infection, anabolic in fixing loose teeth, reduces sensitivity of teeth like sensodent and also ensures oral hygiene." [16]

Many people begin oil pulling to whiten teeth and prevent tooth decay, but then experience the pleasant side effects of more strongly rooted teeth and relief from minor tooth pain... the kind that you may experience when drinking an ice cold or piping hot beverage or biting down on something hard and crunchy.

The reason that oil pulling has this curative effect on teeth has to do with the detoxification and restorative process described in previous chapters. While the toxins are being pulled away and nutrients are added, the tissues around the tooth become healthier and better able to regenerate.

Thus, they begin to heal themselves naturally! What Ayurvedic practitioners seem to know, and western medicine often misunderstands, is that the body strives toward balance and optimal health. When we remove road blocks and give it support, it will get there naturally.

KATE EVANS SCOTT & DAVID PEARSON

4

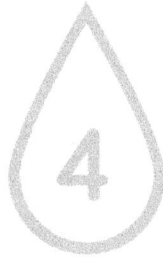

OIL PULLING FOR GENERAL HEALTH

In 1996, an Indian daily newspaper called *Andhra Jyoti* conducted a survey aimed at discovering the effectiveness of oil pulling on health and wellness. Eighty-nine per cent of the 1041 respondents reported that they were cured of one or more diseases with the use of oil pulling in their wellness regime[17]. This newspaper article went viral and kicked off a renewed global interest in the ancient practice of oil pulling already common in India.

Related by Dr. Sarah Larson on her popular health and wellness website, the breakdown of that revolutionary survey is as follows:

Number of Respondents Experiencing Cure with Oil Pulling

- Pains in the body and problems pertaining to neck and above - **758 cases**
- Allergy and respiratory problems of lungs like asthma, bronchitis etc - **191 cases**
- Skin problems like pigmentation, itching, scars, black patches, and eczema etc - **171 cases**
- Digestive system - **155 cases**
- Constipation - **110 cases**
- Arthritis and joint pains - **91 cases**
- Heart disease and [blood pressure] - **74 cases**
- Diabetes - **56 cases**
- Piles - **27 cases**
- Diseases pertaining to female reproductive system reported by women - **21 cases**
- Diseases like Polio, Cancer, Leprosy, polycystic kidney, neural fibroma, paralysis, etc. - **72 cases**

Out of the over one-thousand responses, only 11% claimed that they experienced no notable changes at all. When you take into consideration that many eager people give up on pulling after just a week because they want instant gratification, or that some people do not swish long enough, it's possible that the 11% that experienced no change can be partially credited to "operator error." But even if that small margin of people truly had no positive health changes from the oil pulling, the odds are still quite high that you will find some kind of relief from this ancient Ayurvedic practice.

While this survey was not conducted by scientists in a controlled environment, we cannot discount this kind of anecdotal evidence when making decisions about our wellbeing... especially since oil pulling is a simple, inexpensive process with no known side effects and real research to back the claims of its antioxidant, detoxifying, and regenerative properties... not to mention *thousands of years* of success within the Ayurvedic medical community.

CARDIOVASCULAR HEALTH

Studies at the School of Dentistry at Italy's *University of Cagliari*, along with research published in the *African Journal of Microbiology Research*, clearly link the reduction of oral bacteria to decrease in inflammatory conditions like cardiovascular disease. [18]

These studies now provide further proof for the link between oral health and heart disease that modern medical professionals have been noticing for years.

Most of the oils used in the practice of oil pulling have an incredible antibacterial property that targets inflammation-causing bacteria like *Streptococcus mutans*, decreasing the input of these toxins into the bloodstream and thus having a positive effect on instances of bacterial diseases. The anti-inflammatory properties inherent in these oils reduces instances of inflammatory disease like heart attack, high blood pressure, and stroke.

MIGRAINE TREATMENT AND PREVENTION

Oil pulling has been prescribed for the treatment and prevention of migraines and chronic headaches in Ayurvedic medicine for thousands of years, but it's just now making headlines as a "new" alternative curative for this painful condition.

A migraine is a severe headache that is often accompanied by nausea and vomiting or sensitivity to light and sound. Sometimes a throbbing pain is only felt on one side of the head.[19] Some migraine sufferers are completely incapacitated during the incident and must seek refuge in a dark, silent room until symptoms subside. Other migraine sufferers can maintain some level of activity during the headache with only mild symptoms. In any case, migraines are incredibly painful and somewhat unpredictable because scientists are still unsure as to their exact cause.

However, migraine sufferers have reported similar triggers for their episodes, including stress, hormone changes, lack of sleep, caffeine withdrawal, exposure to smoke, and food triggers like MSG, red wine, nitrates and nitrites, processed foods, and sweets to name just a few. Just how oil pulling breaks down the chain of events that starts with a trigger and ends with a headache is still unclear, but people who get relief from this simple process swear by it.

One thing is very clear, the triggers leading to migraines are often toxins that we put into our bodies or that we are subjected to in our environment. Think in terms of processed foods, wine, caffeine, and sweets among other environmental toxins that our immune system is constantly battling like chemically based soaps and cleaners, exhaust, and cigarette smoke. When you engage in the process of oil pulling, you extract those toxins from your body through the porous oral cavity, thus eliminating or reducing the possible triggers for migraine or chronic headache.

VISION IMPAIRMENT

In an interview with FoxNews.com, Ayurveda expert Dr. Scott Gerson claims that oil pulling has been used in his practice and within the traditional/alternative medical community to effectively treat and prevent many common disorders including vision impairment.[20] "[It's] used as part the multidimensional treatment of impaired vision" he says. "And used extensively in people with far sightedness."

Because vision impairment can be caused by a host of different issues, it's hard to determine whether or not oil pulling will correct an individual's vision problems. Remember, Ayurvedic medicine is a holistic system that takes many factors into consideration to determine a treatment plan. While oil pulling isn't a blanket remedy for vision issues, there are solid reasons why it could potentially aid in the process of restoring healthy eyesight.

Sometimes the root cause of a vision issue is linked to a chronic inflammatory disease. Since we have already determined that oil pulling reduces inflammation, it's easy to see how the practice could help in healing poor eyesight caused by such inflammation. In other cases, poor vision is caused by infection or toxins in the body. Since oil pulling is primarily a powerful detox program, any bodily issue affected by toxins will experience healing, including the ocular system.

Other times, vision issues are caused by tissue damage. When the body flushes out toxins and begins to absorb nutrients, as it does when oil pulling, tissues will begin to repair themselves naturally as the body works toward achieving balance and optimal health. The cleansed and rejuvenated system should restore the damaged tissue more quickly and effectively when utilizing the oil pulling practice.

BONE AND JOINT SWELLING

Bone swelling is indicated by inflammation caused by fluid buildup in the bone or joints. This fluid building can be painful or sore. The swelling is your body's emergency response to the injured area. The fluid wraps itself around the injury, kind of like you'd wrap fine china in bubble wrap before shipping. That way you can continue some normal body function while it heals without causing further injury. When that area fills with protective fluid, it can feel tight and painful to move. People suffering with bone and joint swelling often experience decreased mobility due to the pain and swelling.

The cause of bone and joint swelling varies widely between individuals and from situation to situation. Swelling can come from a bruised or broken bone, which becomes especially painful if the bone is fractured in a way that causes it to protrude from the skin. This type of break exposes the bone to harmful bacteria, which can then enter the bone and infect the marrow, a condition called edema.

Swelling can also be caused by degenerative diseases like rheumatoid arthritis, autoimmune disorders like lupus, and various forms of bone and cartilage cancer.

Oil pulling can help reduce swelling in affected joints and bones by reducing inflammation, attacking harmful bacteria, and boosting the immune system so that it can help your body heal properly and quickly. Dr. Karach himself found almost immediate relief from what seemed a lifetime of arthritis once he began his regular oil pulling routine. Oil pulling tips the body's balance back toward health.

HORMONE IMBALANCE

Human beings have incredibly complicated physiology. When we talk about "hormones," we have to really understand them in the context of the entire system. Hormones are the messengers between glands and the cells that form the tissues of various organs in the body. They are essentially the communication lines of the body, making everything that needs to happen, happen.

Hormones are also responsible for maintaining the chemical levels in the bloodstream, which helps achieve and maintain balance—also called homeostasis. In Ayurveda, balance within the body is the optimal goal.

When someone experiences a hormone imbalance, this means that the endocrine glands are producing either too much or not enough of a particular hormone. Both genders have the primary endocrine glands, which include the pituitary gland, the thymus, the pancreas, the thyroid, and the adrenal glands. The functions of these glands are as follows:

Pituitary: Called the "master gland," the pituitary gland controls the rest of the endocrine glands. If the master gland suffers, the rest of the endocrine system is compromised.

Thymus: The thymus is located on the neck and controls the production of T-cells, an important building block for a healthy immune system. Particularly active during childhood, if the function of the thymus is interrupted and a low T-cell count results, the body can experience a number of symptoms including asthma, immunodeficiency diseases, puffiness and redness around the eyes, and a severely weakened immune system.

Pancreas: Located across the back of the abdomen, the pancreas controls the digestion and metabolism of food. It also produces the hormones insulin and glucagon, which help regulate blood sugar levels. A number of ailments result in a hormone imbalance involving the pancreas, including diabetes.

Thyroid: The thyroid is a butterfly-shaped gland located at the base of the neck, and it controls the body's metabolism. Thyroid function effects everything from your heart rate to how quickly you burn calories. The two main thyroid imbalances are hyperthyroidism and hypothyroidism. Hypothyroidism can cause very serious health affects including weight gain, depression, infertility, and heart problems.

Adrenal Glands: These walnut-shaped glands sitting atop each kidney produce the powerful hormones testosterone, estrogen, and cortisol. They affect every organ in the body and help our chemistry reach homeostasis when under stress. They have serious implications on the way you think and feel. When the adrenal glands are fatigued, there can be serious negative effects on the digestion and metabolism of fats, carbohydrates, and proteins. There can be gastrointestinal problems, changes in sex drive (especially in post-menopausal women), inability to regulate blood sugar and an unhealthy shift in cardiovascular function.

So, the hormones in our bodies are really important to all-around health and well-being. That much is pretty clear. How does oil pulling help keep all of our hormones in proper balance?

While endocrine disorders can be genetic, often they are caused by infection, disease, injury, or a tumor on the gland itself. While there are many different types of hormone imbalances that can result from an endocrine disorder, the most commonly diagnosed in North America is currently diabetes. Other fairly common hormone imbalance symptoms include hyperthyroidism, depression, weight gain, erectile dysfunction, sleep disturbances, and insomnia.

The previously documented research on oil pulling has established its efficacy in regard to bodily **detoxification.** The mouth, especially the tongue, is the most permeable part of the body. This allows for the easy removal of toxins and bacteria that could potentially cause the gland defects resulting in a hormone imbalance.

But the oral cavity also provides the best possible place for **absorption of nutrients,** such as linoleic acids and other essential fatty acids that help boost the immune system and provide the necessary building blocks of the brain. Why is that important? Because the nervous system and endocrine system work so closely to one another that the combination is often called the neuroendocrine system. [21]

The hypothalamus (of the brain) gives the pituitary gland directives, and then the pituitary gland can either enact those directives or veto them. They have a symbiotic relationship. The two systems talk to one another, function hand-in-hand, and both need the essential fatty acids found in high grade oils for optimal wellness.

While the instances relating the curative effects of oil pulling on hormone imbalance are currently just anecdotal, we can't discount the excitement that people have when they find some relief from their symptoms. And remember, these techniques have been employed for thousands of years in the Ayurvedic system specifically for addressing such hormonal imbalances.

SLEEP PATTERN NORMALIZATION

In a response to a blog about oil pulling on a web site called BA50: Better After Fifty, a woman named Nancy responds to oil pulling naysayers with her success in oral health and in finding deep sleep.

"I did try it for 2 weeks," she says. "My teeth did get whiter and felt very clean. I slept better and had dreams for the first time in a long time, indicating deep sleep."

While the anecdotal evidence mounts, (in fact, it's all over the web) scientists agree that further study into the effects of oil pulling on sleep patterns would benefit the medical community. Why would oil pulling make someone sleep deeper, and dream again?

It could be as simple as a detox. Your body does a lot of restorative work when you're asleep. If your body has less to heal, then you will sleep more soundly and peacefully. Perhaps you had a problem with mucous, sinus infection, swollen adenoids, dry throat, aches and pains, and a number of other bacterial or inflammatory diseases that caused your sleep to be disturbed. Once the oil pulling healed those ailments, you returned to a normal pattern of deep rejuvenating sleep.

Another possibility is in the glands. A healthy endocrine system will help ensure the proper production of melatonin, the hormone that regulates sleep. The nutritive and antioxidant properties of the oils help keep the endocrine system running smooth, perhaps ensuring that the melatonin is telling the body to slip into sleep when you slip into bed.

The body and mind are such intricate machines, if one tiny thing goes out of whack, it can throw off the entire operation. In that same vain, one healing practice can put the whole thing back on again and it becomes a healing cycle. Good sleep leads to better health, and better health leads to better sleep.

MENTAL HEALTH

In alternative medicine, we hear a lot about the mind body connection. Even within the mainstream medical community, doctors and researchers are giving more clout to the connection between our physical body and our mental self.

THE STRESS EFFECT

Have you ever noticed your visceral response to your emotions or state of mental well-being? Maybe you felt sick to your stomach when you found out a loved one was in trouble, or you had a headache when you were under a lot of stress. Perhaps you gained weight when you were depressed, or your eczema cleared up when you went on a restful vacation with your partner.

The mind and body are so intertwined that when you commit to a detoxification process in one, it's bound to positively affect the other. That stress that causes you to be irritable, irrational, and anxious can also cause heart disease and diabetes. Why?

Remember the discussion about hormones? Well, hormones regulate our mental health. When we experience a stressor, our adrenal glands kick into high gear and send out hormones to deal with the situation. But what if there's an imbalance in our adrenal gland? Then it might not kick out the right amount of hormones.

Let's say it kicks out too much cortisol. When the adrenal glands are pumping out cortisol to deal with a stressor, the immune system temporarily shuts down. Yes, the immune system actually stops functioning when you are under stress. So, if you keep pumping out the cortisone at an unhealthy level, your immune system stays shut down all that time. Then guess what? You get sick because the immune system is on lock-down while you are feeling totally stressed out. Perhaps you get a cold, the flu, or maybe something more severe that your immune system had been keeping at bay. Then it all becomes a vicious cycle.

What oil pulling does is boost the immune system by flushing out toxins and bacteria while providing powerful antioxidants and anti-inflammatory agents that can help return the body to balance. When the body is in balance, the glands that regulate hormone production and ultimately control the seemingly involuntary emotions of the mind are restored to health. Thus, healthy body, healthy mind.

Many people who try oil pulling immediately experience a lifting of the common "brain fog." First, your mind is a bit sharper and you start remembering where you put your keys. Next thing you know, you are living a totally revitalized life!

THE DETOX EFFECT

It is probably pretty clear to you now that the main function of oil pulling is to detox your body. This is accomplished by pulling the toxins out through the oral cavity. The immediate effect this detox process has on you depends greatly on your individual constitution. Some people begin pulling and experience nothing but the benefits right from the get go—whiter teeth, stronger gums, mental clarity, and the list goes on.

There are a number of reasons for this, one of which being that they are in optimal health. Another person could experience an array of minor "side effects" from starting the oil pulling process. I hesitate to call them side effects, because they are really indicators that the detoxification process is working!

One of the most common "side effects" is nausea and vomiting. This could occur either because of a heightened gag reflex, or more likely because the oil is pulling out toxins that have an impact on the stomach or other parts of the digestive system.

When your body detoxes, it's not just sucking those little bacteria out of the mouth. It's cleansing all kinds of nasty illness from your body, some of which you didn't even know was there. This is why people often feel worse before they feel better when going through any kind of detox process.

Some common, short-lived side effects that have been reported by people just starting the process of oil pulling are:

- Headache
- Nausea
- Vomiting
- Insomnia
- Fatigue
- Stuffy nose/ sinuses

These symptoms are not necessarily side effects of oil pulling, but indicators that the detoxification is actually working! However, that doesn't make stuffy noses and vomiting pleasant. Fortunately, you can take some precautions to minimize these kinds of unwelcome detox symptoms:

- Drink lots of water. A hydrated body heals more easily and helps to flush out toxins. Make sure to drink pure, filtered water to maximize cleansing.

- Eat more protein. Begin to replace processed foods and sweets with lean protein, fruits and vegetables. Just because you're flushing out toxins doesn't mean you can put more in!

- Add essential oils to the detox that effect the particular symptom, such as ginger oil for nausea. (see list in last chapter)

The good news is that these detox symptoms won't last long, if you have them at all. Hang in there, keep oil pulling, and you'll see that all of that pain is worth all of the gain. Within a short period, all of those toxins will be cleared out and your body will be well on its way to attaining balance.

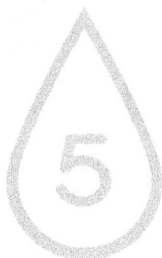

ADDING ESSENTIAL OILS FOR FURTHER BENEFITS

While traditional Ayurvedic oil pulling did little more than possibly add turmeric to the oils, we can now benefit from our extensive knowledge of essential oils for health and wellness to incorporate them into our oil pulling routines.

Some people add a little bit of essential oil, like peppermint or orange, to their base oil when first getting started to help the flavor become more palatable. While this is not always recommended, many new oil pullers have reported that they have experienced no negative effects and have still seen the same results from oil pulling. Just be sure that when you are adding an oil for "flavor," you know that it's a good quality oil, and also know its potential health properties.

Following is a list of essential oils that could be added to your tablespoon of sesame, sunflower, coconut, or olive oil prior to swishing. Remember to just add a small drop, as pure essential oils can have very powerful properties.

ESSENTIAL OILS TO ADD TO PULLING

- **Basil Oil** can refresh the mind and restore you to a more mentally alert state. This is a good one to add for lifting "brain fog."

- **Clove Oil** is an antibiotic, analgesic, and is good for treating the gums and teeth. Use this to help strengthen gums, alleviate swollen tissue, and whiten teeth.

- **Frankincense** is an analgesic, antiseptic, and anti-inflammatory agent. It's good for alleviating sore throat symptoms, removal of warts and skin tags, and centering yourself.

- **Geranium Oil** is a good one to add if you have laryngitis. It also helps strengthen gums and clean teeth.

- **Grapefruit Oil** is a powerful cleansing agent, a good one to add to kick start your detox.

- **Ginger Oil** is a digestive aid that provides relief for upset stomachs. It also has a pleasant flavor with a little kick of spice.

- **Lemon Oil** is a good oil to add if you gag easily and might have the propensity to gag while pulling. It is also a powerful cleansing agent and has a positive effect on sore throats and common cold symptoms.

- **Lemongrass Oil** will help cure herpes.

- **Melaleuca Oil** (or tea tree oil) is antibacterial, anti-inflammatory, and antiseptic. It helps boost the immune system, stave off colds and flu, and alleviate pain from orthodontics and mouth sores. The flavor, however, is a little bit piney and does not sit well with every palate.

- **Nutmeg Oil** is soothing. It has a calming affect while also boosting the nervous and endocrine systems. This might be a good supplemental oil if you are experiencing hormonal imbalance.

- **Oregano Oil** is a powerful multipurpose essential oil that effectively combats influenza (the flu), common cold, symptoms of a sore throat, and swollen glands. It is antibacterial, antibiotic, antiviral, and has anti-inflammatory properties.

- **Peppermint Oil** soothes upset stomachs and has a pleasant taste that could help alleviate gagging while pulling.

- **Sage Oil** helps support several body systems including reproductive, nervous, and respiratory systems. It boosts metabolism and can also help with mental fatigue.

If you're going to try out essential oils, remember to use baby steps. You're starting out a whole new detox routine. Don't also introduce your body to a new essential oil. Start with an oil you've used effectively in the past.

GET STARTED

Setting aside the fact that oil pulling has been in use for thousands of years, or that there are now numerous accounts from people all over the world who can confirm the validity of this practice, the simple truth of the matter is that oil pulling deserves more than our passing interest.

If offering up just 15 minutes a day (and yes of course, that can still be a lot for some of us!) is all we need to reap the health benefits of this practice, then what are we waiting for? If you live in the USA where health care is privatized, then it only makes sense that we explore the great healing potential of this tried and tested alternative practice. After all, purchasing a container of coconut oil or (whatever oil you prefer) is a small price to pay compared to the lengthy medical bills some of us are so used to seeing!

Whether your goal is to whiten your teeth and freshen your breath, or the issues go deeper, oil pulling is such a simple and inexpensive healing therapy that you can't help but give it a try! Put a bottle of your chosen oil and a spoon or small cup (like a shot glass) next to your bathroom sink. Take a shot and swish. It's that easy. Honestly, the minutes go by quickly and you'll start to look forward to the meditative time in the morning. Don't get frustrated after a few days... results take between one and two weeks. But once you start seeing the positive changes in your smile, and in your health, you won't want to stop pulling.

The advice in this book is not intended to replace professional medical attention. Always consult your physician when beginning a new medical practice, especially if the goal is to target a specific medical condition. Do not discontinue taking prescribed medication without consulting your physician.

RESOURCES

1) McClernon FJ1, Yancy WS Jr, Eberstein JA, Atkins RC, Westman EC. The effects of a low-carbohydrate ketogenic diet and a low-fat diet on mood, hunger, and other self-reported symptoms. Obesity (Silver Spring). 2007 Jan;15(1):182-7.
http://www.ncbi.nlm.nih.gov/pubmed/17228046

2) Seaton TB, Welle SL, Warenko MK, Campbell RG. Thermic effect of medium-chain and long-chain triglycerides in man. Am J Clin Nutr. 1986 Nov;44(5):630-4.
http://www.ncbi.nlm.nih.gov/pubmed/3532757

3) Gunnars, Kris. Top 10 Evidence-Based Health Benefits of Coconut Oil. Authority Nutrition. 8 July 2013
http://authoritynutrition.com/top-10-evidence-based-health-benefits-of-coconut-oil/

4) Olive Oil, Extra Virgin. The World's Healthiest Foods. Whfoods.com http://www.whfoods.com/genpage.php?tname=foodspice&dbid=132

5) Sunflower Oil. Fitness Republic.
http://www.fitnessrepublic.com/nutrition/fats-oil/sunflower-oil.html

6) Ayurveda-History & Philosophy. Traditional and Indigenous Healing Systems. Healthy and Healing in NY.
http://www.healthandhealingny.org/tradition_healing/ayurveda-history.html

7) Chopra, Deepak, MD. What is Ayurveda? Chopra Centered Lifestyle. 16 March 2013
http://www.chopra.com/ccl/what-is-ayurveda

8) Singh, Abhinav and Bharathi Purohit. Tooth brushing, oil pulling and tissue regeneration: A review of holistic approaches to oral health. J Ayurveda Integr Med. 2011 Apr-Jun; 2(2): 64–68.
http://www.ncbi.nlm.nih.gov/pmc/articles/PMC3131773/

9) Vasant Lad, B.A.M.S., M.A.Sc. Tongue Analysis. The Ayurvedic Institute.
http://www.ayurveda.com/online_resource/tongue_analysis.html

10) Asokan S1, Emmadi P, Chamundeswari R. Effect of oil pulling on plaque induced gingivitis: a randomized, controlled, triple-blind study. Indian J Dent Res. 2009 Jan-Mar;20(1):47-51.
http://www.ncbi.nlm.nih.gov/pubmed/19336860

11) The Tooth Decay Process: How to Reverse It and Avoid a Cavity, National Institute of Dental and Craniofacial Research. http://www.nidcr.nih.gov/OralHealth/OralHealthInformation/ChildrensOralHealth/ToothDecayProcess.htm

12) Asokan S, Kumar R S, Emmadi P, Raghuraman R, Sivakumar N. Effect of oil pulling on halitosis and microorganisms causing halitosis: A randomized controlled pilot trial. J Indian Soc Pedod Prev Dent 2011;29:90-4
http://www.jisppd.com/article.asp?issn=0970-4388;year=2011;volume=29;issue=2;spage=90;epage=94;aulast=Asokan

13) Gingivitis. A.D.A.M. Medical Encyclopedia. PubMed Health. Reviewed 22 February 2012.
http://www.ncbi.nlm.nih.gov/pubmedhealth/PMH0002051/

14) (10)

15) Amith, Dr. HV, Anil V Ankola, L. Nagesh. Effect of Oil Pulling on Plaque and Gingivitis. JOHCD Jan 2007; 1 (14) http://www.johcd.org/pdf/Effect_of_Oil_Pulling_on_Plaque_and_Gingivitis.pdf

16) http://www.oilpulling.com

17) Oil Pulling: What the Wise Ones in India do Almost Every Day. http://drsarahlarsen.com/organic-health/oil-pulling/

18) Wright, Carolanne. Oil pulling: A cheap, easy and effective solution to health woes? Modern research says yes. 12 May 2013. http://www.naturalnews.com/040293_oil_pulling_cognitive_decline_home_remedies.html#

19) Migraine. A.D.A.M. Medical Encyclopedia. PubMed Health. 2 November 2012 http://www.ncbi.nlm.nih.gov/pubmedhealth/PMH0001728/

20) Grush, Loren. What is oil pulling? Examining the ancient detoxifying ritual. Fox2News. 24 March 2014 http://www.foxnews.com/health/2014/03/24/what-is-oil-pulling-examining-ancient-detoxifying-ritual/

ABOUT THE AUTHORS

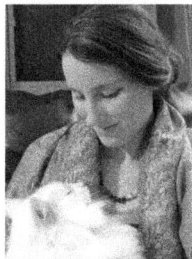

KATE EVANS SCOTT is the author of the Amazon Bestselling cookbooks The Paleo Kid, Paleo Kid Snacks, The Paleo Kid Lunchbox and Infused: 26 Spa-Inspired Natural Vitamin Waters.

After her son was diagnosed with several food intolerances and after having struggled with her own Autoimmune Disease, Kate made the commitment to remove all grains and processed foods from her family's diet. Her passion and love for good food blossomed after training with a retreat chef in Belgium in her early 20's. Since then, she has wanted to bring her love of food and health into the kitchens of other families struggling with health and dietary challenges.

Kate creates delicious dishes that are suitable for those suffering from digestive and autoimmune diseases - meals that nourish the body while healing the gut. Kate and her husband Mark live in Oregon with their two spirited children.

DAVID PEARSON has over 10 years experience in emergency and survival training from the oil and gas industry. He left his field after witnessing the startling devastation and impact that drilling is taking on our planet, its communities and natural resources.

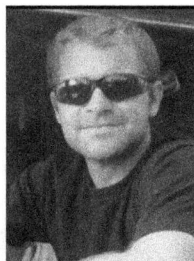

His greatest passion is being outdoors and learning new ways to tread lightly. He lives on a homestead in Oregon with his wife, two children and his dog Ernie.

MORE BY KATE & DAVID

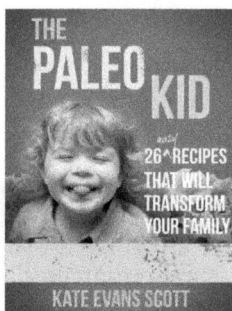

Available Now on Amazon

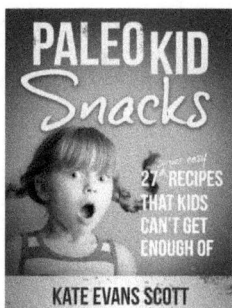

Available Now on Amazon

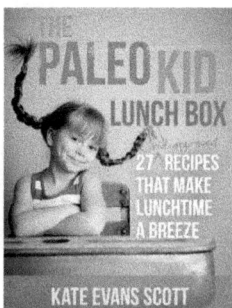

Available Now on Amazon

MORE BY KATE & DAVID

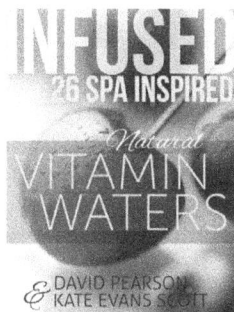

Available Now on Amazon

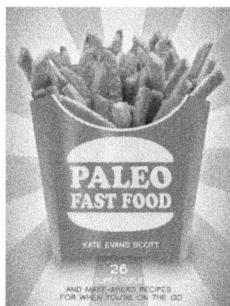

Available Now on Amazon

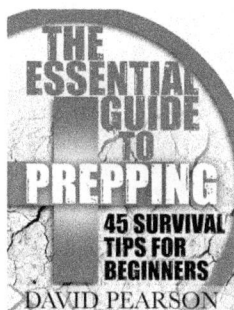

Available Now on Amazon

VISIT:

www.KidsLovePress.com

FOR MORE GREAT TITLES ON

HEALTHY LIVING!!

KATE EVANS SCOTT & DAVID PEARSON